Kick your Butts Goodbye Forever

How Electric Acupressure Will Help you Quit Smoking for the Last Time

Written by

James P. Seim, DC, DACBN
Diplomate American Clinical Board of Nutrition

First Printing, 2018

ISBN 9-781987-796445

Allied Health Professions - Chiropractic
Alternative Medicine - Acupuncture & Acupressure
Addiction and Recovery - Smoking

Corcoran Hamel Chiropractic PA
James P. Seim, DC, DACBN
20010 75th Ave N
Corcoran, MN 55340
WWW.Quit2Live.com

.

"I used to take a puff from my dad's cigarette in the ash tray."

"My dad died from a heart attack when I was five."

—Jim Seim

For a short video presentation please go to my website:

www.quit2live.com

There you will find a description of the program with the current cost and inclusions in the program.   Your investment in the program is less than the cost of one pack of cigarettes a day for one month in my home State of Minnesota.

Contents

Introduction

Let's face the fact that quitting smoking is one of the more difficult undertakings you will take in your life. It is also one of the most rewarding. I would like you to accept this as an invitation to change your life. Thousands of individuals since 1980 have become nicotine-free with the help of this program, and yes, it can help you. This book is primarily for those individuals who are able to personally take advantage of my in-office treatment in my home State of Minnesota. This is the ideal approach to personally commit to your new, nicotine-free life.

The first and most difficult aspect of breaking the nicotine addiction is making the decision to quit. The fact that you are reading this book means you are like most people addicted to nicotine, you want to quit, you are just not sure how. You know it is not good for you. In addition to being socially unacceptable, there is a substantial expense involved. We will be discussing in great detail the fact that smoking, vaping, or chewing are not instinctive behaviors, but something you learned how to do. It did not take long to learn but once you did, it quickly became a habit. This book will show you how to unlearn the behavior and forever break that habit.

During withdrawal from nicotine you may experience the following symptoms; nervousness, irritability, knots in the stomach, and the feeling of climbing the walls. These are the aspects where my program of electronic acupuncture truly excels at controlling the symptoms. With my program, there will be a change in the electrical and chemical impulses flowing in your body. It is definitely a strange experience. In the office, we deal with the electrical changes. On your own, at home, you deal with the chemical changes. You will also continue to use the powerful, yet simple technique I teach to help you break the habit.

My expertise so far has been helping those inside of an office setting. That is the focus of this book.

The Habit Poem

I am your constant companion. I am your greatest helper or heaviest burden. I will push you onward or drag you down to failure. I am completely at your command. Half of the things you do you might as well turn over to me and I will do them—quickly and correctly. I am easy to manage—you must be firm with me. Show me exactly how you want something done and after a few lessons, I will do it automatically. I am the servant of great people, and alas, of all failures as well. Those who are great, I have made great; those who are failures, I have made failures. I am not a machine, though I work with the precision of a machine plus the intelligence of a person. You may run me for profit or run me for ruin—it makes no difference to me. Take me, train me, be firm with me, and I will place the world at your feet. Be easy with me and I will destroy you. Who am I?

I am Habit.

—Author Unknown

Can You Break the Addiction?

"It is hard to understand addiction unless you have experienced it."

—Ken Hensley

If I can quit, you can quit!

I honestly do not remember when I had my first cigarette. I used to sneak a puff of my dad's L&Ms when they were burning in the ashtray. He died from a heart attack when I was only five years old. I continued to smoke throughout my school age years. The only time I ever quit smoking was for 2 years in grade school.

When I entered chiropractic college, smoking was still socially acceptable; there was a smokers' lounge at the college. In the following four years of intense training in natural and holistic health care you would think my education as to the devastating effects of smoking would be enough to make me stop. Never underestimate the ability to rationalize. I was young and healthy and could quit whenever I wanted. In fact, I never bought a carton of cigarettes as I was always going to quit after this pack. There was one exception to this rule; whenever I was going on vacation, the first thing I would pack is a carton of cigarettes. There was no way I would ever quit on vacation! By the time I was an intern, smokers were banished to the parking lot outside. In the middle of January in St. Paul, Minnesota, it could easily have been 10 to 20 degrees below zero actual air temperature and I would be out there, puffing away on my Old Gold Lights.

I was truly a nicotine addict having smoked for 35 years. Eventually the price had to be paid for the sins of my youth. In 2015 I suffered a heart attack and underwent an emergency quadruple coronary artery bypass graft.

I know your nicotine addiction and exactly what you are going through, having been there many times. I am truly on your side. I want you to succeed as a non-smoker. Together lets spare you from future health challenges.

A Twist of Fate

"Men are not prisoners of fate, but only prisoners of their own mind."

— Franklin D. Roosevelt

In 1980, I went on an Oriental study tour to observe acupuncture in China. It was the experience of a lifetime: 12 full days inside China, observing everything from Mao's Mausoleum to the Great Wall and the Pandas at the Peking Zoo. The highlight of the trip was to observe a surgery using acupuncture anesthesia. What an experience!

When I returned from China, a patient called me. She had heard of a chiropractor using acupuncture to help people quit smoking. She asked if I could do the procedure for her. I was unaware of the procedure, but I told her I would investigate and get back to her.

I tracked down a chiropractor in northeast Minneapolis who was doing the smoking cessation procedure using electronic acupressure. He was kind enough to share the formulae and I called my patient, Patty, to give it a try. To our amazement, it worked wonderfully! Patty soon became my greatest promoter.

Patty was a flight attendant for Northwest Orient Airlines and she shared her success with other flight attendants across the country. Soon they were knocking at my door form New York, California, and Washington State. They were flying in, non-revenue, for this amazing treatment. Note: I had not yet "taken the cure" myself.

My reputation continued to spread by word of mouth, one person at a time. On July 21, 1982, the front page article above the fold of the Canby News, a small town on the border of Minnesota and South Dakota, featured a local resident, Sharon Birk who had come to my St. Paul office and gone through the program with great success. She had been a 25-year smoker, up to two packs daily. It was quite a nice article and extremely accurate with respect to the description of my program, even though I had not been interviewed and was only referred to as a "Saint Paul chiropractor." The referrals from South Dakota soon started streaming in.

On September 29, 1982, a top-ranking official in the Minnesota National Guard came for the treatment. He had smoked three to four packs of cigarettes per day for nearly 40 years. He was also one of my greatest successes. The referrals from the Guard exploded. I had so many green uniforms coming in the door; I think he might have been ordering people to quit. Who knows—maybe he was!

The program spread by word-of-mouth and I kept getting busier and busier. I had no real formal training in the program and had been flying by the seat of my pants, but the astounding thing was it worked. On average, two out of every three people forever rid themselves of their nicotine addiction. I would follow up with them in 30 days and again, after about one year. One of the more interesting items I noticed when following up with the people was that rarely did they consider the program a failure. Rather, they complimented the way it had worked for them, and they tended to blame their own shortcomings when they found some excuse to go back and become a smoker all over again. Let's face it, smokers look for excuses.

In 1989, the local Coca Cola distributor made the decision to go smoke-free as a company. Since many of their employees had been in the program successfully, they made a corporate decision to offer their employees the program at the company's expense. Soon, there were 10 to 25 employees coming in every week. I was spending 45 minutes to an hour going over the program and losing my voice in the process. By necessity, I needed a short cut to the program, and the video was born. The edited transcript of the video is the next chapter. It describes in detail what is necessary to quit smoking and why the electronic acupressure works so well.

What Are You Going to do, Doc?

"Desire is the starting point of all achievement, not a hope, not a wish, but a keen pulsating desire, which transcends everything."

—Napoleon Hill

I am going to discuss my procedure to help you quit smoking. The procedure is electronic acupressure. There are no needles, I do not break the skin, and it does not hurt. While it is strange, it is not painful.

What it is designed to do and what it will do for you is to decrease your physiological desire for nicotine. In other words, you will not crave cigarettes. You should not be irritable, feisty, nervous and headachy. You also should not experience knots in the stomach or be climbing the walls. These are the types of sensations it will take care of. What is doesn't do and what I need to teach you to do is to deal with the psychological or habitual aspects. For example, when you get into the car, pick up the phone, enjoy a cup of coffee, have a cocktail - whenever you habitually reach for a cigarette.

What you need to understand is that smoking is a learned behavior - not instinctive, but rather, learned behavior. Since you learned it, you can unlearn it. Take a moment to drift back in time, before you had your first cigarette. There was no pleasure associated with smoking and there was no pain associated with not smoking. It was the most normal, most natural, and most instinctive way to be.

When you had your first cigarette, it was a painful experience. You coughed, you gagged and you turned a little green. However, in a short period of time, you learned to associate cigarettes with pleasure and not smoking with pain. That is one of the reasons why so many people have trouble ridding themselves of the habit. They associate cigarettes with pleasure and not smoking with pain. It is not instinctive, but a learned behavior and you can unlearn it or re-educate yourself. The way to unlearn it is to associate cigarettes with pain and not smoking with pleasure.

The way to accomplish this is *every time—and I do mean every time*—you think of cigarettes or you unconsciously start to reach for a smoke, you need to have a physical gesture that causes you some degree of pain. You will need to either slap your hand or put a rubber band around your wrist and snap it.

Your thoughts should be that cigarettes are pain, cigarettes: pain, cigarettes: pain. Repeat this over and over again! Replace the thought of having a cigarette with "I am happy. I am healthy and my lungs are clear!" Repeat this affirmation as often as possible.

I know it seems simple, but it is powerful. It will help break the habit if you perform it. It will not do any good do not. My statement is "it's like exercise and prayer; it will not help if you do not do it."

What you need to remember is that the tobacco industry has literally spent billions—and I mean *billions* of dollars—to try to control your mind to make you do something that is instinctively harmful, intellectually disgusting, and physically debilitating. And guess what? They have won! You are addicted to nicotine and cigarettes.

Additives are placed in the tobacco to "enhance flavor" and these additives increase the addictive nature of their product to even a greater extent than nicotine alone. In addition they have associated cigarettes with everything positive, everything pleasant, everything sexy, and they have planted it deep into your subconscious mind. If you are old enough you may remember the old phrase "Winston tastes good like a (clap clap) cigarette should." The federal government forced that off the air in 1971. You have not heard that for decades. If you do not remember this, or if you are not old enough, you are responsible for your own physiological indoctrination.

Whenever you have a pleasant experience, an emotional set back, been happy, sad, grieving, celebrating, been nervous or when you are relaxed you have shared all those experiences and more with a cigarette. You reached for the cigarette, sat back, and reflected on those experiences. The cigarette has become your best buddy. Now, when you find yourself nervous or uptight, you reach for a cigarette thinking that it will relax you.

In reality, cigarettes are a stimulant. They do not relax you, and you cannot smoke a cigarette when hunched over. In order to smoke a cigarette, you have to change your posture and physiology. You must bring your shoulders back, hold your head high, and take a deep breath or drag. This posture feels much more comfortable. If you do catch yourself getting nervous or uptight, you can change your posture and physiology directly. Just bring your shoulders back, hold your head high, take a deep breath, and say, "Ahhh I have traded cigarettes for breathing and it feels terrific."

Another thing that affects a vast majority of patients going through the program is that prior to the age of six, one or both of their parents have smoked cigarettes. Even if this does not apply to you read on. You need to understand that before the age of six, you do not have the ability to discern what is right or wrong. Your brain is literally in programming mode. You just assume that everything your parents do is correct or "God-like". They may have told you, "Don't smoke cigarettes," but 20 times a day they showed you it is okay to smoke…it is okay to smoke…it is okay to smoke, and you have that programming in your subconscious mind.

The tobacco industry has also done a great deal of unconscious programming, along with all of your good and negative experiences and what your parents have likely also done. You could spend thousands of dollars and years of therapy to try to undo it piece by piece, or you can bypass that mechanism. This is the power behind slapping your hand or snapping a rubber band. This is when you must repeat the affirmation: "I am happy, I am healthy, and my lungs are clear!" Use the rubber band or slap your hand—there is a real power in it. I know that it seems silly, but if you use it, it will work. The nice thing is, if you no longer physically crave cigarettes after this program and you use this technique, it makes it easier to break the habit. This is the way I describe the program. Nobody can make you quit, but I can make it easier for you to quit.

This is where the electronic acupressure comes in. What will take place within your body is an actual electrical and chemical change. I am going to physically and temporarily change the way electricity flows in your body.

This is a very powerful psychological tool called a pattern interrupt. There are nine different points that are stimulated electrically. When I apply the electrical acupuncture, your muscles will contract in harmony with the electrical impulses. Stimulating the ninth acupuncture point on the lung meridian—located on the wrist—causes the hands to move in harmony with the impulses. It is not painful; rather, it is usually quite humorous. One of my patients, Ray, called that particular maneuver the "flopping crappie". It is psychologically a powerful tool that will leave you with a lasting pattern interrupt.

Later we will discuss how on your own, at home, you are going to change your body chemistry with some dietary changes.

What is really going to happen to me?

You are likely wondering what changes are taking place inside your body because of the electronic acupuncture? Your brain naturally secretes chemical substances called neurotransmitters, which controls the way you think, act and feel. The ones we are going to discuss today are endorphins, serotonin and dopamine. While this is not meant to be a course in neurophysiology you need to understand some of the concepts. Bear with me while I explain a few of the basic principles. Endorphins are natural pain killers that activate opiate receptors. They are also responsible for the "runners high" reported by marathon athletes. Serotonin is the happiness hormone. Depression patients are treated with drugs called SSRI's or selective serotonin reuptake inhibitors expecting an increase in serotonin will increase happiness. Dopamine is the pleasure hormone. Dopamine is responsible for addictive behaviors. The difference, however, is dramatic and has been blurred by cleaver marketers for the years. They would like you to believe their product, that provides pleasure, is actually providing happiness.

According to Dr. Robert H. Lustig, M.D. Retired Professor of Pediatrics, Division of Endocrinology University of California, San Francisco; "Pleasure is short-lived, visceral, usually experienced alone, achievable with substances. Happiness, by contrast, is often the opposite—long-lived, ethereal, and often experienced in social groups and cannot be achieved through substances. Pleasure is taking, while happiness is giving. Pleasure relies on dopamine, while happiness relies on serotonin. These emotions involve two very different neurotransmitters, regulatory systems and pathways in the brain."

Nicotine stimulates the dopamine receptors in your brain to give you pleasure, which is short lived and leaves you with the sensation of craving another dose of nicotine. The electronic acupuncture will reset your dopamine receptors. As long as you do not stimulate these receptors with nicotine, you will not crave more nicotine. Break down and have one puff of a cigarette and your dopamine receptors be reactivated and you will crave more. You will go back and smoke just as much as if not more to make up for the time your receptors were feeling deprived.

As a side note, Sean Parker, the founder of Napster and first president of FaceBook, is quoted "We need to sort of give you a little dopamine hit every once in a while, because someone liked or commented on a photo or a post or whatever... It's a social-validation feedback loop... a vulnerability in human psychology."

These changes to the neurotransmitters are the physical reality. It is helpful if you imagine a meridian system or channel of energy inside your body. Imagine it like a garden hose with water or a life force flowing through it. Then imagine is that over a period of time, smoking has clogged these channels with nicotine. What I do for you, in one fell swoop, is to blast those channels clear. As long as they are clear ***and they stay clear***, you should not have the desire to smoke.

That leaves us with a word of caution: this is not the type of thing where you can say to yourself "I will just have one cigarette—it won't hurt." It will! You will clog up those channels, your dopamine receptors will shout "that's what I have been missing." You will go through withdrawal again. If that happens, I do not consider that a failure, instead know I am on your side; I want you to succeed as a non-smoker. I will provide at no additional cost a second treatment within six months.

As a former smoker, you will look for an excuse to go back and have that first cigarette. Someone will cut you off in traffic and you will raise your fist and say, "I'll show you! I am going to have a cigarette." Do you think the other driver really cares? You may be in a boat with a buddy and he lights up a cigar and you think that it looks pretty good and it is not really smoking, is it? It is! It is like being pregnant—you are or you are not, there is no in-between. Either you are a smoker or you are not a smoker. Have you ever woken up and said to yourself: "I wish I never would have started that filthy habit?" Well, you have that opportunity right now.

Of all the things there are to do on this entire planet, there is only one choice you have to commit to. It is not that you can't smoke, because you can. Rather it is your choice to not put the very first cigarette into your mouth and light it. If you do not have the first puff of a cigarette, one day at a time, you will be a non-smoker, it's as simple as that. It's also as hard as that.

Never tell yourself, your friends or your family that you are "trying" to quit smoking. Using the word "try" is excusing failure in advance. "I am going to try but I am not going to make it!" Instead you **have** quit smoking.

You may be asking yourself: what are some of the things I should expect from the program? There are two very separate and distinct components to the program. The first is the physiological effects of addiction and that is very powerful. I have had recovering alcoholics and drug addicts tell me it was harder to give up cigarettes than it was to give up alcohol or heroin.

The other aspect is the psychological addiction. Ten years from now, when you have not had a cigarette in that entire time, there will be some unknown trigger anchored deep in your subconscious and you will all of a sudden say to yourself, "Jeez, I can't believe it—I just craved a cigarette." It will pass and pass very quickly, but that's how powerful psychological addiction is. Soon, we will be discussing a very simple yet very powerful technique that will make it easier for you to break the psychological or habitual addiction.

However, as physiologically addictive as nicotine is, the physical addiction will be over and done within 21 days. Three weeks from now, when you have not had a cigarette, the physical withdrawal will be over and done and you will no longer be addicted to nicotine. Most people in the program are amazed that the first two and half weeks are remarkably simple, then, about day 18, 19, or 20 their bodies go through this little flip-flop and screams at them, "Are you sure you want to do this to me?" That will be your final withdrawal from nicotine.

Once you have made it through the withdrawal at three weeks, the next challenge will be at your one-month anniversary. You may have a tendency to feel confident as you pat yourself on the back and think to yourself, "This has been one of the easiest times I have ever had quitting smoking. I'm going to celebrate. I'm going to have just one cigarette and then quit all over again." Don't do that. You cannot have just one cigarette. What you are doing, instead, is making a conscious decision to go back and be a smoker all over again, as much as before, and maybe even a little more to make up for lost time.

Dietary Considerations

Let's discuss the chemical changes that are going to take place inside your body. These are actually dietary considerations that you'll be taking care of on your own at home.

I want to go over this point-by-point, so you will know exactly what to expect. When your body chemistry is more acidic, you tend to crave cigarettes; when your body chemistry is more alkaline, you will not crave cigarettes. Now, the first thing on my list seems to contradict this: I want you to find a natural source of vitamin C. You need to eat two citrus fruits daily. I prefer that you eat the fruit rather than drink the juice. When you eat the fruit, your blood sugar does not spike as high when compared to drinking the juice, and your body will convert the acid to an alkaline ash in your lungs. Do not go overboard with the fruit—limit yourself to two a day. I have had people call me up to say they have just had their fourteenth orange and they are going nuts—what is going on? The answer is that you are acidic and you will crave cigarettes. Since you are taking a natural source of vitamin C, do not take a vitamin C supplement—most vitamin C products are pure ascorbic acid and will acidify your body, making you crave cigarettes.

If you take a multi-vitamin, please check the vitamin C content. If it is 60 mg or less feel free to continue the vitamin. However, you may need to increase intake of the mineral water I am going to talk about shortly. If your vitamin has more than 60 mg of vitamin C, hold off for the next three weeks or so, depending on how easy it is going for you.

The next thing on our list is green vegetables. Please eat at least one green vegetable per day. More is better. Green means green: lettuce, broccoli, spinach or green beans—whatever you prefer; you cannot eat too much. If you are looking for a snack, I strongly recommend sunflower seeds. Get the ones that are still in the shell. This serves two purposes. First, they give you something to do with your hands, keeping them occupied, and second, they will alkalize your body. Do not get the ones that are already shelled as you will tend to grab handfuls which has the tendency to support weight gain, and I do not want you to gain weight on the program. As a matter of fact, one out of three people actually lose weight on the program, one out of three maintains their weight within one to three pounds, and about one-third tends to gain weight. This is why I want you to get unshelled sunflower seeds.

The next two things on the list are the most important things I will ask you to do. Please do the following: drink at least one bottle of mineral water every day. Perrier, San Pellegrino, Klareblun, H_2O, and Mendota Springs all produce mineral water. If you cannot find mineral water, club soda will work—any brand you like is fine. What will not work are flavored waters with sugar, high fructose corn syrup, or artificial sweeteners such as Splenda (which is Sucralose) or NutraSweet (which is aspartame). These will acidify your body, causing you to crave cigarettes. If you do find a product that is sweetened exclusively with stevia, it will likely be acceptable.

Mineral water has that funny, bubbly taste. You do not have to drink a full bottle—four ounces is all you need to knock out a craving in moments. Your state will immediately change. It works! Get some today. Keep it with you at home, at work, and the office. If you do not like the taste, it is still essential to take advantage of the benefits of mineral water! Stop on the way home and get the mineral water. If you do nothing else that I talk about, the mineral water will help. If you are experience cravings, you may drink two, three, four, five, even six bottles of mineral water. If you drink two or more bottles, be aware it is a natural diuretic which flushes out your system, and that is good. **Get the mineral water.**

Do not replace cigarettes with candy or sweets. A lot of folks meet their downfall when they "try to quit smoking" and go cold turkey. They go out and by a bag of Tootsie Pops, put them on their desk, and when they have a craving take the candy instead. Candy is extremely acidic and it makes you crave cigarettes even more. These people grab a piece of candy and want a cigarette even more, so they grab another piece of candy and another piece of candy and another piece. They do this for three days, gain five pounds, and say, "This is ridiculous. I want a cigarette worse than ever." So they go back smoking to try to lose the weight they put on. Don't do that!

Do NOT replace cigarettes with candies or sweets. Now, if you have dessert after dinner, it is okay. Be aware, you may experience a craving, slap your hand or use the rubber band and it will pass.

Next on the list is to avoid alcohol. It is not forbidden—you may drink, but the more you avoid it the easier it will be for you. It is the most common reason people require a second treatment. Following a drink or two, your judgment becomes impaired and you associate drinking with smoking. In addition alcohol is extremely acidic. It is a triple whammy—if you are going to have a drink, it is okay, but you need to make a conscious decision before your first drink that you are going to keep in control, that you will not let that little, white cigarette rule your life, that you are in control. After a drink or two, you may say to yourself: "What the heck—one smoke won't hurt me." IT WILL. If you have a cigarette while you are drinking, you will likely buy a package that night, smoke the majority of the pack, wake up the next morning with your lungs aching, and you will feel terribly, terribly guilty.

Finally, avoid red meat. Following a heavy meal of red meat, your body pours in stomach acid which changes your body chemistry making you acidic. The acid also breaks down the protein in the meat releasing nitrogen byproducts into your system. Remember your last steak or prime rib. You thought, "AAHH! I can't wait for that cigarette—it is going to taste so good!" That was due to the chemical changes in your body.

Eggs and poultry, especially turkey, are good alternative sources of protein as they contain the amino acid tryptophan, the precursor of the neurotransmitter serotonin, which promotes the "feel good" or happiness factor in your brain.

Other than these two times, you should be like the majority of people who come into the office here. I do not know what the Doctor did to me—black magic or what. You see, it is remarkably simple: you have already quit smoking. I just need to make certain, one day at a time that you do not start again.

At this point in time, I ask if there are any questions and if there are not, we can go to work. The next step is to stimulate the acupuncture points with my electronic muscle stimulator. I will stimulate nine points on your body to begin with.

The first step is to celebrate your birthday!

Congratulations! You are a non-smoker. Of all the things there are to do in this universe, there is only one thing you must choose not to do, and that is to put the first cigarette in your mouth and light it. It is that simple. It is that hard. Exercise your new found freedom from nicotine.

If you do have any difficulties, the first thing to do is to slap your hand or use the rubber band. Cigarettes equal pain…cigarettes…pain. I know it seems simple and silly. It is powerful and it works. The next thing is to drink the mineral water—four ounces will knock out a craving in moments. If you still have problems, give me a call. Frequently, we can work it out on the phone. Other times, you will need to come in for another treatment. If you do, currently there is no charge for an additional treatment within the next six months.

As a former smoker you may still look for an excuse to have that first puff of a cigarette. My wife, Kerry, works in the office me. She is a former smoker, as well. She also enjoys giving our patients her advice. She urges patients to learn how to do nothing. Smokers use cigarettes as an excuse to take some time for themselves. You need to understand that you have the power and the freedom to choose to do nothing and relax all on your own, without a cigarette. Look for a mentor who does not smoke and model their behavior.

The Beginning of your Smoke-Free Life

"We are what we repeatedly do. Excellence, then, is not an act, but a habit."

—Aristotle

Day 1: Do not smoke. Do not put the first cigarette into your mouth and light it. You have the freedom and the power to say NO to the very first cigarette. If you do not put the first cigarette in your mouth and light it, none of the others will ever be a problem. Remember to slap your hand or use the rubber band. I know it seems silly or dumb but it works. Drink the mineral water.

Day 2: Do not smoke. Do not put the first cigarette into your mouth and light it. You have the freedom and the power to say NO to the very first cigarette. Remember to slap your hand or use the rubber band. Drink the mineral water.

Day 3: Do not smoke. Do not put the first cigarette into your mouth and light it. Remember to slap your hand or use the rubber band. Drink the mineral water.

Day 4: Do not smoke. Do not put the first cigarette into your mouth and light it. Remember to slap your hand or use the rubber band, Drink the mineral water.

Day 5: Do not smoke. Do not put the first cigarette into your mouth and light it. Remember to slap your hand or use the rubber band, Drink the mineral water.

Day 6: Do not smoke. Do not put the first cigarette into your mouth and light it. Remember to slap your hand or use the rubber band, Drink the mineral water.

Day 7: Congratulate yourself on a successful week. I expect you should be feeling good about your decision by now. Remember: do not smoke. Do not put the first cigarette into your mouth and light it. Remember to slap your hand or use the rubber band, Drink the mineral water.

Day 8: Do not smoke. Do not put the first cigarette into your mouth and light it. Remember to slap your hand or use the rubber band, Drink the mineral water.

Day 9: Do not smoke. Do not put the first cigarette into your mouth and light it. Remember to slap your hand or use the rubber band, Drink the mineral water.

Day 10: Do not smoke. Do not put the first cigarette into your mouth and light it. Remember to slap your hand or use the rubber band, Drink the mineral water.

Day 11: Do not smoke. Do not put the first cigarette into your mouth and light it. Remember to slap your hand or use the rubber band, Drink the mineral water.

Day 12: Do not smoke. Do not put the first cigarette into your mouth and light it. Remember to slap your hand or use the rubber band, Drink the mineral water.

Day 13: Do not smoke. Do not put the first cigarette into your mouth and light it. Remember to slap your hand or use the rubber band, Drink the mineral water.

Day 14: Celebrate your second week and congratulate yourself for two weeks of success. It was, indeed, a wise decision. Do not smoke. Do not put the first cigarette into your mouth and light it. Remember to slap your hand or use the rubber band, Drink the mineral water.

Day 15: Start to be more careful. Your body is close to being nicotine-free. You may be feeling confident but your body is going through the final stages of withdrawal, so please remember: you have the power and freedom to say NO. Remember: it is like being pregnant—either you are or you are not; there is no in-between. Do not smoke. Do not put the first cigarette into your mouth and light it. Remember to slap your hand or use the rubber band, Drink the mineral water.

Day 16: Continue with caution. Do not smoke. Do not put the first cigarette into your mouth and light it. Remember to slap your hand or use the rubber band, Drink the mineral water.

Day 17: By now you should understand there are only a few things you need to do to be a permanent non-smoker. Do not smoke. Do not put the first cigarette into your mouth and light it. Remember to slap your hand or use the rubber band, Drink the mineral water.

Day 18: If today is a little tough, celebrate—your body is working through its physical addiction to nicotine. Do not smoke. Do not put the first cigarette into your mouth and light it. Remember to slap your hand or use the rubber band, Drink the mineral water.

Day 19: It should be getting a little easier today. Do not smoke. Do not put the first cigarette into your mouth and light it. Remember to slap your hand or use the rubber band, Drink the mineral water.

Day 20: Do not smoke. Do not put the first cigarette into your mouth and light it. Remember to slap your hand or use the rubber band, Drink the mineral water.

Day 21: Celebrate! Your nicotine addiction is physically over with, however, do not get to confident. Psychologically, the addiction will last for the rest of your life. Ten years from now, when you haven't had a cigarette in all that time, something will inevitably trigger the thought to have a cigarette. Don't worry—it will pass very quickly. Do not smoke. Do not put the first cigarette into your mouth and light it. Remember to slap your hand or use the rubber band, Drink the mineral water.

Day 22: Do I really need to keep repeating this? Do not smoke. Do not put the first cigarette into your mouth and light it.

Remember to slap your hand or use the rubber band, Drink the mineral water.

Day 23: Do not smoke. Do not put the first cigarette into your mouth and light it. Remember to slap your hand or use the rubber band, Drink the mineral water.

Day 24: Do not smoke. Do not put the first cigarette into your mouth and light it. Remember to slap your hand or use the rubber band, Drink the mineral water.

Day 25: Do not smoke. Do not put the first cigarette into your mouth and light it. Remember to slap your hand or use the rubber band, Drink the mineral water.

Day 26: Do not smoke. Do not put the first cigarette into your mouth and light it. Remember to slap your hand or use the rubber band, Drink the mineral water.

Day 27: Do not smoke. Do not put the first cigarette into your mouth and light it. Remember to slap your hand or use the rubber band, Drink the mineral water.

Day 28: Happy Four-Week Anniversary! The instructions have not changed. Do not smoke. Do not put the first cigarette into your mouth and light it. Remember to slap your hand or use the rubber band, Drink the mineral water.

Day 29: Do not smoke. Do not put the first cigarette into your mouth and light it. Remember to slap your hand or use the rubber band, Drink the mineral water.

Day 30: You are now one month smoke free! Hurrah! Do not start patting yourself on the back, thinking this was one of the easiest times you have ever had quitting smoking. Do not celebrate and think you can have just one cigarette and then quit all over again. DO NOT DO THAT! Do not make a conscious decision to go back and start smoking all over again.

I hope you have found this information beneficial in your quest to improve your life and your health. I look forward to hearing about your success.

You may contact me with compliments or concerns at DrJimSeim@gmail.com   Website is www.Quit2Live.com

A final thought: "I am not telling you it is going to be easy- I am telling you it is going to be worth it."   Art Williams